IMPACT OF VARIOUS ACTIVITIES DURING PREGNANCY

HINAL PATEL

Contents

Preface   *v*

Acknowledgements   *vii*

  1. Introduction   1

  2. Effect Of Mantra/music   4

  3. Effect Of Yoga, Meditation, Light Exercise   16

  4. Diet Counselling And Prenatal Education   34

  5. Art Based Activity   47

  6. Bibliography   50

Preface

Pregnancy is a very special and important time in a woman's life, in which the mother-to-be prepares herself for her new role as a mother. Concepts of Garbhasanskar and it's need in current scenario, Physical and mental purification before inception, Role of parenting to develop child's personality and IQ, Need for healthy and safe Pregnancy, Proper Conception along with great soul invitation from universe to mother's womb etc. The literal meaning of Garbhsanskara is educating the fetus in the womb. It is a way of teaching good things to unborn baby in womb during pregnancy.

The advantages of Garbhasanskara are not only that you educate your child and there is development of a bond between the mother and the child. In fact, this has a great impact on the health of the mother also. The positive thinking and attitude promotes physical well-being of the mother.

This book has been written keeping in mind the importance of different activities which has to be done during pregnancy. The information contained within is review of latest research findings in a simplified yet exhaustive manner to benefit one and all.

We earnestly hope that readers will enjoy reading the book and benefit from it and also spread the valuable information among those around them.

Hinal Patel

May, 2022

Acknowledgements

Acknowledgement is due to the Vice-Chancellor Shree Harshad P. Shah, Children's University, Gandhinagar who gave their valuable comments and inputs.
Special thanks to the Registrar Dr. Ashok Prajapati, Children's University, Gandhinagar for the support and encouragement in accomplishing the task.
I thank Dr. Rakesh Patel for the encouragement, motivation and joy he has for this work.

CHAPTER ONE

INTRODUCTION

The children's are the creator of bright future. Physically healthy, radiant in mind and intellect, generous by heart and full of inner strength, such children will become the best citizen of the Nation and they will create the Great Nation of Twenty-First century. For such holistic development of the children Hon'ble Chief Minister of Gujarat Shri Narendra Modi has established Children's University which ensures to provide all needed help and care for the integral development of the Child and Tapovan is its first step towards this new endeavor which would provide Prenatal Care and Education. Because Child education must begin at prenatal stage and education must continue right through the whole life. Thus the expectant mothers have a very unique role to play in this progress of human evolution.

Becoming a mother is the most important phenomenon in a woman's life and childbirth is the most precious event. Thus a pregnant woman has to be given special care throughout the pregnancy to ensure the perfect health of her baby and herself which is rightly done with SUPRAJA – a complete protocol for maternal care. Ayurveda recognized the need for the mental, spiritual and physical preparation of the mother-to- be for the momentous event of childbirth. It involves the preparation of the couple planning pregnancy, three months prior to conception. Ahara (diet), Vihara (lifestyle), Sadavrutta (moral conduct), along with varied therapies give wonderful results. Along with normal nutritious diet, specific diets for each month of Antenatal period depending on embryogenesis. Diets with specific impact on the fetus, specifically effective on reproductive & endocrine systems.

The concept of 'Tapovan', introduced by Children's university has been formulated taking into consideration the integral development of fetus by revitalizing and strengthening the mother's aspiration to give birth to a soul who will be a fore-runner of a New humanity in an age when the people are under a strong influence to achieve materialistic fulfilment rather spiritual fullness.

Tapovan has been conceptualized taking into consideration the modern life style of the people. Tapovan will provide an opportunity to pregnant woman to devote herself not only for her self-development, but also to the growth of the fetus taking place within her body because the woman's role is that of a mini creator. So, it is natural for her to feel happy as she is forming a baby within. Motherhood is the happiest moment for any woman. There are many aspects which influence the women, when she is pregnant. During pregnancy many activities have been carryout by Tapovan centre:

1. Mantra/ singing stuti/ rhymes/music
2. Yoga, pranayam, light exercise
3. Diet counselling
4. Prenatal Education and Counselling
5. Story telling

6. Art and Craft

CHAPTER TWO

EFFECT OF MANTRA/MUSIC

Playing music

The latest data shows that music and language are so intertwined that an awareness of music is critical to a baby's language development. As children grow, music fosters communication skills. Our sense of song helps them to learn to talk, read, and even make friends. A study of musician's brains shows in excess of five times as many interconnections in the brain than non-musicians. Student musicians have an average of 11 points higher IQ than non-musicians.

Effects of Music

These effects are instant and long-lasting. Music is supposed to link all the emotional, spiritual, and physical elements of the universe. Music can also be used to change a person's mood, and has been found to cause physical responses in many people simultaneously.

On Body

It decreases the blood pressure and enhances the ability to learn. Music affects the amplitude and frequency of brain waves, which can be measured by an electroencephalogram. Music also affects the breathing rate and electrical resistance of the skin.

On Mind

As the body becomes relaxed, the mind is able to concentrate more easily. The simultaneous left and right brain action maximizes learning and retention of information. Students' listening skills also improved through music education. Musical training has an effect on how the brain gets wired for general cognitive functioning related to memory and attention. It is clear that music is good for children's cognitive development and that music should be part of the preschool and primary school curriculum. It helps in improving learning and neuroplasticity; neuroplasticity is the brain's ability to repair connections and form new neural connections (wiring) in response to a new situation. A study of the brains of musicians shows in excess of 5 times as many interconnections in the brain than non-musicians. Student musicians have an average of 11 points higher IQ than non-musicians

On Relationship

Music enhances prenatal bonding. One of the most intimate and pleasurable events experienced by the baby in the womb is his mother's singing. It is also one of the first dialogues exchanged between mother and child. Songs that communicate love, acceptance, and welcome are most reassuring to the baby. This is a two-way process whereby the mother and child form a close attachment, developing trust, a feeling of safety and a sense of belonging. All other relationships will depend on the quality of this first exchange. If we are nurtured lovingly with and consistency, then we will most likely to treat others in the same manner.

Music Therapy

Music and sound are beginning to play an active role in medicine as evidenced by studies in neurobiology and psychology. In this regard, music therapy is also making a contribution to the healing arts.

Benefits of Listening to Music on Mother

1. It improves the bonding between the mother and the baby.

2. She is able to come out of stress and overcome the physical ailments or complications, if any, and handle pregnancy confidently.

3. Makes the mother relaxed and feel less pain during labour and aids in normal delivery.

Benefits of Listening to Music on Baby after Delivery

1. Womb song is like a lullaby, makes a crying baby stop and puts it to sleep.

2. Helps in taking breast-feeding better.

3. There is heightened awareness in these babies after birth and they smile and talk early and easily.

Listening to music if continued after delivery, helps babies talk early and have superior language skills. It also improves mathematical skill and communication skill. The heartbeat of the mother is the first familiar rhythm for the baby. Heart beat plays the major part of reassurance and, as per Dr. Verny, it acts as a major life support system in the world of babies. Dr. Verny terms a mother's heartbeat lovingly and rightfully as the "Womb Music."

That's why when mother or anyone lulls the baby by placing it on the left side of the chest close to heart, the baby hears again the familiar rhythm and calms down and falls asleep soon.

Various experiments have shown that plants exposed to classical music all day, thrive and grow well. On the other hand, plants exposed to heavy metal music all day shrivelled up. Heavy metal music had a very definite negative impact on plants. Although this doesn't mean that it will have the same negative effect on your baby, heavy metal music is not soothing, either for the mother or for the baby, and as such, it will certainly have no positive impact on your child. In addition, beats are random rather than rhythmic, and sudden shifts in volume may startle your child. Religious music and mantras impart positive vibrations and are a good idea. Stick to a mix of classical, pop and religious music and chants.

Music can help calm your baby, as your baby will find it easier to identify beats, and rhythmic sounds work well with babies. However, also remember that a baby's breathing pattern changes according to beats, and listening to pounding music with rapid beats for an extended period may stress out your baby.

1. **Author**: Pithadiya, A. C., Makwana, D., & Tomar, S.

Title: Garbhasanskar - A Technique of Educating Foetus Yoga During Pregnancy

Journal: *Pharma Science Monitor*, 2016, 7(1), 50-56

The ancient scriptures and Ayurveda prescribe music and mantras to be listened to during pregnancy. The sound of the veena (Indian string instrument which is held by the Goddess Saraswati) and the Samaveda mantras also give health to the pregnant woman and the child within. It is possible to give energy for the development of the body, mind and soul of the child in the womb by listening to special music. The important qualities of leadership, bravery, creativity and love for all can be cultured in the child by listening to specific composition.

1. **Authors:** Agrawal, T., & Gupta, P. K.

   Title: Garbha sanskar – A boon to get supraja
   Journal: *The Pharma Innovation Journal, 7(6), 454-456.*
   It is proved that fetus also responds to the mantra/ music. From 7th month fetus can hear the sounds from mother's womb and from the surroundings of mother and also responds to them. Sound of mother's heartbeats is the first and nearest sound heard by the fetus and hence when the mother takes her crying child close to her the child stops crying and becomes calm. It is possible to give energy for the development of body mind and soul of the child in the womb by listening to special music. The sound of the veena (Indian string instrument which is held by the Goddess (Saraswati), flute and Samaveda mantras gives health to the pregnant woman and the child within.

   Chanting of mantra like Vanshvriddhi Vanshkavach Stotra, Garbha rakshan Prarthana and Garbha rakshan Sookta, Gayatri mantra and Pragya vivardhan stotra etc.- These are musical interpretations of essential mantras and stotras that create an environment of spiritual tranquility and learning for the mother and child and they also helpful in mental health and brain development of child.

3. **Authors:** Wulff, V., Hepp, P., Wolf, O. T., Balan, P., Hagenbeck, C., Fehm, T., & Schaal, N. K.

   Title: The effects of a music and singing intervention during pregnancy on maternal well-being and mother–infant bonding: a randomised, controlled study
   Journal: *Archives of gynecology and obstetrics, 2021, 303(1), 69-83.*

Stress and impaired mother–infant bonding during pregnancy can lead to adverse effects for the expectant mother and the unborn child. They studied the effects of a music and singing intervention during pregnancy on maternal well-being and mother–infant bonding. Methods A total of 172 pregnant women took part in this prospective, randomised, three-armed (music, singing or control group) study. Depressive symptoms, self-efficacy, maternal well-being and mother–infant bonding were assessed with visual analogue scales and questionnaires before the intervention phase (30th week of gestation) and afterwards (36th week of gestation). Additionally, immediate changes regarding experienced stress and mood from before until after the music and singing interventions were explored with questionnaires as well as saliva samples (for cortisol, alpha-amylase and oxytocin determination). Results Regarding immediate effects, both interventions showed positive effects on the emotional state, stress (cortisol) and bonding (oxytocin). Additionally, the singing group showed a larger reduction in cortisol and a larger improvement in valence than the music group. Looking at more prolonged effects, significant effects on general self-efficacy and perceived closeness to the unborn child (measured with a visual analogue scale) were found. No significant effects were revealed for the mother–infant bonding questionnaire and for depressive symptoms. They conclude that prenatal music and singing interventions could be an easy to implement and effective addition to improve mood and well-being of the expectant mother and support mother-infant bonding.

4. **Authors**: Chang, M. Y., Chen, C. H., & Huang, K. F.

Title: Effects of music therapy on psychological health of women during pregnancy

Journal: *Journal of clinical nursing*, 2008, *17*(19), 2580-2587.

This controlled study demonstrated that a prescribed two-week regimen of music therapy significantly reduced the intensity of stress, anxiety and depression in pregnant women. Music therapy is a cost-effective, enjoyable, non-invasive therapy and could be useful in creating an environment that is conducive to the well-being of the pregnant women.

5. **Authors**: García González, J., Ventura Miranda, M. I., Requena Mullor, M., Parron Carreño, T., & Alarcón Rodriguez, R.

Title: Effects of Prenatal Music Stimulation on State/ Trait Anxiety In Full-Term Pregnancy and Its Influence On Childbirth: A Randomized Controlled Trial

Journal: *The journal of maternal-fetal & neonatal medicine*, 2018, *31*(8), 1058-1065.

It can be said that the non-stress test procedure is anxiogenic, and that listening to music during this procedure has a positive impact on pregnant women by reducing their degree of anxiety. The use of prenatal music stimulation with relaxing and instrumental music over a period of fourteen 40-minute music sessions may be beneficial and effective as a tool to reduce anxiety in full-term pregnant women during an non-stress test, while helping them to relax, and as a result improve the delivery process by reducing the first stage of labor in nulliparous women.

6. **Authors**: Nwebube, C., Glover, V., & Stewart, L.

Title: Prenatal listening to songs composed for pregnancy and symptoms of anxiety and depression: a pilot study

Journal: *BMC complementary and alternative medicine,* 2017, *17*(1), 1-5.

Pregnant women were recruited online and randomly assigned to one of two groups: the music group (daily listening to specially composed songs) or control group (daily relaxation) for 12 weeks each. Self-report questionnaires were used to assess symptoms of State and Trait anxiety (Spielberger) and depression (Edinburgh Postnatal Depression Scale (EPDS)). Trait anxiety was measured as the primary outcome, while State anxiety and depression were the secondary outcomes. 111 participants were randomised to each group. 20 participants in the intervention group and 16 participants in the active control group completed the study. Results: The music group demonstrated lower Trait Anxiety (p = .0001) (effect size 0.80), State Anxiety (p = .02) (effect size 0.64), and EPDS (p = .002) (effect size 0.92) scores at week 12 compared to baseline, by paired t test. There were no such changes in the control group. Conclusions: Though this pilot study had high levels of attrition, the results do suggest that regular listening to relaxing music should be explored further as an effective non-pharmacological means for reducing prenatal anxiety and depression.

7. **Authors**: Akmeşe, Z. B., & Oran, N. T.

Title: Effects of Progressive Muscle Relaxation Exercises Accompanied by Music on Low Back Pain and Quality of Life During Pregnancy

Journal: *Journal of midwifery & women's health*, 2014, 59(5), 503-509.

Back pain is commonly experienced by pregnant women. Evidence suggests that progressive muscle relaxation (PMR) therapy, a complementary therapy widely used by pregnant women, may improve the physical and psychological outcomes of pregnancy. The aim of this study was to investigate the effects of PMR training accompanied by music on perceived pain and quality of life (QOL) in pregnant women with low back pain (LBP). This was a prospective randomized controlled trial. The study was designed to examine the effects of PMR accompanied by music on pregnant women with LBP. In total, 66 pregnant women were assigned randomly to a PMR group or a control group (33 women in each). A personal information form was used as a data collection tool; a visual analog scale was used for measuring pain; and the Short Form-36 was used to evaluate QOL. The control and intervention groups were comparable at baseline. Significant differences were observed between the 2 groups after 4 and 8 weeks of intervention. The intervention group showed significant improvement in all QOL subscales after the intervention. The intervention group, but not the control group, showed significant improvement in perceived pain after the intervention. The intervention group experienced a greater decrease in perceived pain and improved QOL than the control group. DiscussionOur findings show that PMR accompanied by music may be an effective therapy for improving pain and QOL in pregnant women with LBP.

8. **Authors**: Chang, H. C., Yu, C. H., Chen, S. Y., & Chen, C. H.

Title: The effects of music listening on psychosocial stress and maternal—fetal attachment during pregnancy
Journal: *Complementary therapies in medicine*, 2015, *23*(4), 509-515

The effectiveness of music listening in helping pregnant women cope with stress, especially pregnancy-related stress. Although this study found no effect for music listening on either general perceived life stress or maternal—fetal attachment, the evidence indicates that music is an effective, non invasive pregnancy-related stress intervention for women that has minimal or no side effects and is cost effective and convenient. These findings have significant implications for healthcare professionals who wish to incorporate this safe non-pharmacological intervention into prenatal care. This intervention program can be sustainable and can be tailored and promoted to enhance relaxation and maternal—fetal attachment.

9. **Authors**: Arya, R., Chansoria, M., Konanki, R., & Tiwari, D. K.

Title: Maternal Music Exposure during Pregnancy Influences Neonatal Behaviour: An Open-Label Randomized Controlled Trial
Journal: *International journal of pediatrics, 2012.*

This study provides preliminary evidence that maternal music exposure beneficially affects neonatal behaviour. A trained clinician can utilize the behavioural organization of the newborn infant to gain insights into the intrauterine experience and the perinatal events which may have influenced the neonate's central nervous organization. The present clinical trial was not designed to study these aspects and provides no information regarding the mechanism behind the observed effect. Further studies should confirm this observation with a more rigorous design and try to elucidate the direct and endocrine-mediated mechanisms of the effect of music on foetus and newborn.

10. **Authors**: Fritz, T. H., Ciupek, M., Kirkland, A., Ihme, K., Guha, A., Hoyer, J., & Villringer, A.

Title: Enhanced response to music in pregnancy
Journal: *Psychophysiology*, 2014, *51*(9), 905-911.
Given a possible effect of estrogen on the pleasure-mediating dopaminergic system, musical appreciation in participants whose estrogen levels are naturally elevated during the oral contraceptive cycle and pregnancy has been investigated (n = 32, 15 pregnant, 17 nonpregnant; mean age 27.2). Results show more pronounced blood pressure responses to music in pregnant women. However, estrogen level differences during different phases of oral contraceptive intake did not have any effect, indicating that the observed changes were not related to estrogen. Effects of music on blood pressure were independent of valence, and dissonance elicited the greatest drop in blood pressure. Thus, the enhanced physiological response in pregnant women probably does not reflect a protective mechanism to avoid unpleasantness. Instead, this enhanced response is discussed in terms of a facilitation of prenatal conditioning to acoustical (musical) stimuli. In conclusion, they observed an enhanced physiological response in pregnant women in terms of systolic and diastolic blood pressure

during the perception of musical stimuli and its spectrally and temporally modified counterparts. For all participants, they observed the same valence-independent pattern of response, where dissonantly manipulated music (but not comparably unpleasant music played backwards) led to a decrease in blood pressure. Such an enhanced physiological response in pregnant women could potentially facilitate prenatal musical conditioning.

11. **Authors**: Surucu, S. G., Ozturk, M., Vurgec, B. A., Alan, S., & Akbas, M. **Title**: The effect of music on pain and anxiety of women in labor during their first pregnancy: A study from Turkey

Journal: *Complementary therapies in clinical practice*, 2018, *30*, 96-102.

This study aims at analyzing the effect of music on pain and anxiety felt by women in labor during their first pregnancy.When the pregnant women in the experimental group progressed into the active phase of the labor, they were made to listen to music in Acemasiran mode with earplugs for 3 hours (20 minutes of listening with 10-minute breaks).It was observed that after the first-hour women indicated that their pain was statistically less in the experimental group. Trait anxiety scores of the women in labor were similar for experimental and control groups. Following the practice, state anxiety average scores became lower in favor of the experimental group and the correlation was statistically significant. They **concluded that in** order to facilitate women's coping with labor pain and improve their wellbeing with the activity during the labor, musicotherapy, a non-pharmacological method, is an effective, simple and economical method.

CHAPTER THREE

Effect of Yoga, Meditation, Light Exercise

Yoga in pregnancy is multi dimensional physical, mental, emotional and intellectual preparation to answer the challenges faced by a pregnant woman. The challenges of pregnancy are revealed by the state of happiness and stress while *yoga* is a skill to calm down the mind. Pregnancy in a woman is a condition in which woman changes both from inside as well as outside. These changes create obstacles or hurdles in the normal life of a pregnant woman and *yoga* in pregnancy can help the women to cruise through these changes and challenges.

Practicing *yoga* during pregnancy provides a great range of activity and benefits to unborn child and mother by numerous ways. *Yoga* soothes the mind, refocus the energy and prepare the woman physiologically and psychologically for labour. Different breathing techniques impart invaluable neuro-muscular control and helps in coordinated relaxation and contraction of uterus. Different type of *asanas* (postures),are described in *Ayurveda* and *Yoga darshan* texts which can be performed by a pregnant woman as they consume low energy and provide greater benefits.

Published articles and different studies with references have been considered to support the effect of *yoga* in pregnancy. *Yoga* practicing includes physical postures and breathing techniques which minimizes the complication of pregnancy, like pregnancy induced hypertension, intrauterine growth retardation and pre-term delivery etc. Western exercises bring about what is known as phase contraction of muscles while yogic exercises create a static contraction which maintains a muscle under tension without causing repeated motions. An approach to *yoga* in pregnancy can improve birth weight; decrease pre-term labour, decreased IUGR with least or no complications.

Padmasana

Butterfly Pose or Titali Asana-This asana opens up your hips and inner thighs, and removes tension from the inner thigh area. In addition, it stretches your knees and groing area. It is one of the most beneficial pregnancy poses and if done consistently right from the first trimester, it will almost certainly ease childbirth to a great extent

Squats or Utthanasan- This is similar to the position adopted by housecleaners when they sweep the floor, which is why sweeping floors is actually excellent exercise.

Cat Stretch Pose or Marjari Aasana - This Aasans strengthens your neck, shoulders and spine, which is why it is also very good for the posture. In addition, it tones up the entire reproductive system, and is very beneficial for women before, during and after pregnancy.

The benefits of Yoga Asanas

- Relieves fluid retention which can be common in the last months.
- Influences the position of the baby and turning it in advance if need.
- Strengthening and massaging the abdomen helps stimulating bowel action and appetite.
- Raises the level of energy and helps in slowing down the metabolism to restore focus.
- Helps in reducing morning sickness, nausea and mood swings.
- Relieves tension around cervix and birth canal.
- Focuses on opening the pelvis to make labor easier and quicker.
- It helps in post natal care -it restores the uterus, abdomen and pelvic floor
- Also it relieves upper back tension and breast discomfort after delivery.
- It restores body shape after childbirth.

Meditation
There are different types of meditation
Mindfulness meditation is a form of meditation where you focus on the physical and emotional sensations that are going on in the present moment without judging how they make you feel.

Transcendental Meditation involves repeating a mantra silently.

Heartfulness meditation is focusing on heart. They have a special program for expecting mothers. The heartfulness institute in association with IAP has formed "Mission Lakshya 1000." It believes in providing nutrition with nurturing environment in the critical period of first 1000 days starting from preconception through pregnancy up to two years of life. They associate themselves with the pregnant mother in her journey, helping her to maximize the child's potential, there by the nation's future.

Walking meditation is a kind of meditation where you walk mindfully for a fixed amount of time. You may choose to focus on your breath or your steps.

Deep breathing is one of the most effective ways to ease muscle tension, lower heart rate and help fall asleep. It requires the expecting mother to breathe deeply and rhythmically. Breathe slowly through nose for four seconds, keeping the mouth closed. Be conscious of stomach rising as you gradually fill the lungs and diaphragm with air, then hold for one second before exhaling through the nose to the count of four. It can be done at anytime and in any posture.

Body scanning is a form of progressive relaxation that involves sitting or lying down while focusing on various parts of the body and breathing into those places of tension that need to be released.

Progressive muscle relaxation technique, which includes body scanning meditation, may take a couple of weeks to master. It's like a natural sleeping pill, which we'll really appreciate as pregnancy progresses and a good night's sleep becomes more and more elusive. Here's how to do it: Lie down on the bed or on the floor and tense the muscles completely...then let them totally relax. Focus on one muscle group at a time and alternate between the left and right side of your body. One possible route is to start by tensing and releasing the hand and forearm muscles, followed by the triceps and biceps, then the face, the chest and shoulders, stomach, legs and finally, the feet

Guided imagery or visualization.

Just picture yourself in a place you find peaceful or relaxing- a tropical beach, a flower-filled meadow or wherever your own private bliss may be. Next, imagine every detail of that place, from the sounds to the smells and everything in between. An alternative to this technique is to think of an image from a magazine or photograph and fill in every detail in your mind Visualization takes some practice, but once you get it, you'll find it's a great way to quieten your mind, ease your tension and help you drift off to sleep.

When done consistently over an extended period of time, meditation can have a host of positive benefits physical and mental to the expectant moms. There are many benefits, both physical and mental both to mother and the baby, Scientific studies have proven the efficacy of yoga and meditation in pregnancy.

1) Meditation can help with pregnancy symptoms, including fatigue, mood changes and sleep disturbances.

2) Studies have found that meditation and other mindfulness-based exercises during pregnancy reduce anxiety, perceived stress.

3) It helps in reducing post-delivery depression.

4) It removes fear and pain associated with childbirth. It reduces perceptions of the pain and length of labor.

5) Body awareness can also be vital in helping pregnant women notice early on if something doesn't feel quite right, like leaking of amniotic fluid and decrease in fetal movement. This helps in taking treatment early which may be a very crucial step in preventing serious complications for the mother and the baby.

6) Yoga and meditation significantly improve birth weight, prevent premature births, and reduce medical complications for the mother and the baby.

1. **Author**: Pithadiya, A. C., Makwana, D., & Tomar, S.

Title: Garbhasanskar - A Technique of Educating Foetus
Journal: *Pharma Science Monitor*, 2016, 7(1), 50-56
They said breathing techniques and meditation also helps in developing positive thoughts and will make you feel well from within.

1. **Authors**: Chaudhary, I., & Joshi, B.

Title: Efficacy of Blessings Meditation as a Behavioral Medicine in Enhancing Pregnancy Happiness
Journal: *Age (years)*, 20(25), 18.
Behavioral medicine is a tool of psychology applied to health and medicine. Conventionally, underlying negative emotional and psychological states that may produce pathological physiological consequences and social consequences gain attention, contradictory to them, positive emotional state of happiness is a way of enhancing health and wellbeing. Everyone is in pursuit of happiness; meditation is a tool for reaching the source of eudaimonic happiness, the authentic happiness that comes from self-actualization. Pregnancy is equalized to self-actualization in psychologically healthy mothers, on the other hand it is also counted as major life stressor that requires adjustment. The study aims at enhancing the positive appraisal of their pregnancy among pregnant women through blessings meditation as a behavioral medicine tool. The present study is a pre test-post test study with comparison group, 60 pregnant women who gave consent to participate in the research were divided into two groups, control (N=30) and experimental (N=30). Experimental group was given blessings meditation intervention for 12 weeks. Degree of

pregnancy happiness was assessed using Pregnancy Happiness Scale. Blessings meditation has proved to be efficient as a behavioral medicine in enhancing pregnancy happiness of the pregnant women.

3. **Author**: Pithadiya, A. C., Makwana, D., & Tomar, S.

Title: Garbhasanskar - A Technique of Educating Foetus
Journal: *Pharma Science Monitor*, 2016, 7(1), 50-56

Although it may sound strange and weird, your bond with your child starts right from the time you conceive. It is not that when the child is born you know him. The baby listens to you and feels your feelings even when it is developing in your womb. You can shape up your baby's first impressions by listening to good music, visualizing, massaging gently meditating and of course, with the help of positive thinking.

4. **Authors**: Beddoe, A. E., Yang, C. P. P., Kennedy, H. P., Weiss, S. J., & Lee, K. A.

Title: The Effects of Mindfulness-Based Yoga During Pregnancy on Maternal Psychological and Physical Distress
Journal: *Journal of Obstetric, Gynecologic & Neonatal Nursing*, 2009, 38(3), 310-319.

To examine the feasibility and level of acceptability of a mindful yoga intervention provided during pregnancy and to gather preliminary data on the efficacy of the intervention in reducing distress. Baseline and post-treatment measures examined state and trait anxiety, perceived stress, pain, and morning salivary cortisol in a single treatment group. Post intervention data also included participant evaluation of the intervention. The 7 weeks mindfulness-based yoga group intervention combined elements of Iyengar yoga and mindfulness- based stress reduction. Sixteen healthy pregnant nulliparous women with single ton pregnancies between 12 and 32 weeks gestation at the time of enrollment. Outcomes were evaluated from pre- to post intervention and between second and third trimesters with repeated measures analysis of variance and post hoc nonparametric tests. They found women practicing mindful yoga in their second trimester reported significant reductions in physical pain from baseline to post intervention compared with women in the third trimester whose pain increased. Women in their third trimester showed greater reductions in perceived stress and trait anxiety.

5. **Authors**: Chuntharapat, S., Petpichetchian, W., & Hatthakit, U.

Title: Yoga during pregnancy: Effects on maternal comfort, labor pain and birth outcomes

Journal: *Complementary therapies in clinical practice*, 2008, *14*(2), 105-115.

A randomized trial was conducted using 74 primigravid Thai women who were equally divided into two groups (experimental and control). The yoga program involved six, 1-h sessions at prescribed weeks of gestation. A variety of instruments were used to assess maternal comfort, labor pain and birth outcomes. The experimental group was found to have higher levels of maternal comfort during labor and 2 h post-labor, and experienced less subject evaluated labor pain than the control group. In each group, pain increased and maternal comfort decreased as labor progressed. No differences were found, between the groups, regarding pethidine usage, labor augmentation or newborn Apgar scores at 1 and 5 min. The experimental group was found to have a shorter duration of the first stage of labor, as well as the total time of labor.

6. **Authors**: Tejwani, N., Roy, P. K., & Mishra, R.

Title: Role of Yoga for Better Outcome Of Pregnancy

Journal: *National Journal of Integrated Research in Medicine*, 2013, 4(4),12-15.

Group of 50 women taking antenatal care were included in the study, a questionnaire was designed to assess the effect of regular Yoga exercises, on the mode of labour and outcome. They found that regular yoga exercises and follow up had a positive impact on results regarding outcome improvement and reduced complication rate. They concluded that regular yoga exercises gives an opportunity to create a world for the baby that is healthy and peace full by coordinating movement, breath and awareness, addresses health and wellbeing on several levels: physical, emotional, psychological and spiritual. Because of its many benefits, yoga is becoming increasingly accepted everywhere as part of self-care during pregnancy and preparation for childbirth and motherhood.

7. **Authors**: Dhapola, M. S., & Prasad, M. R. K.

Title: Role of Different Asanas during Prenatal and Postnatal Pregnancy

Journal: *International Journal of Physical Education and Sports*, 2018, 3(12), 9-16.

Yoga may be beneficial and there are plenty of benefits of asana for physical and mental health to tackle the unbearable pain of pregnancy leading efficient delivery of the baby. Increase one's overall performance, health, and quality of life. If practicing yoga regularly; we can serve a peaceful, healthy life and work without any hindrance. With the help of Yoga, you can tackle any tricky situations may face by women during prenatal and postnatal pregnancy. asana may be assist the women about increasing stamina, strength, reducing pain, depressive symptoms, anxiety, improve recovery time, encourage good posture, create space in growing uterus and preparing mind for labor.

8. **Authors**: Narendran, S., Nagarathna, R., Narendran, V., Gunasheela, S., & Nagendra, H. R. R.

Title: Efficacy of Yoga on Pregnancy Outcome
Journal: *Journal of Alternative & Complementary Medicine*, 2005, *11*(2), 237-244.
Three hundred thirty five (335) women attending the antenatal clinic at Gunasheela Surgical and Maternity Hospital in Bangalore, India, were enrolled between 18 and 20 weeks of pregnancy in a prospective, matched, observational study; 169 women in the yoga group and 166 women in the control group. Women were matched for age, parity, body weight, and Doppler velocimetry scores of umbilical and uterine arteries. Yoga practices, including physical postures, breathing, and meditation were practiced by the yoga group one hour daily, from the date of entry into the study until delivery. The control group walked 30 minutes twice a day (standard obstetric advice) during the study period. Compliance in both groups was ensured by frequent telephone calls and strict maintenance of an activity diary. Birth weight and gestational age at delivery

were primary outcomes. They found the number of babies with birth weight ≥ 2500 grams was significantly higher ($p < 0.01$) in the yoga group. Preterm labor was significantly lower ($p < 0.0006$) in the yoga group. Complications such as isolated intrauterine growth retardation (IUGR) ($p < 0.003$) and pregnancy-induced hypertension (PIH) with associated IUGR ($p < 0.025$) were also significantly lower in the yoga group. There were no significant adverse effects noted in the yoga group. They concluded that an integrated approach to yoga during pregnancy is safe. It improves birth weight, decreases preterm labor, and decreases IUGR either in isolation or associated with PIH, with no increased complications.

9. **Authors**: Gupta, A., Janu, N., & Punia, R

Title: Efficacy of Yoga & Anupreksha in Natural Birthing and Reducing Labor Duration

Journal: Journal Of Humanities And Social Science (IOSR-JHSS), 2018, 23(4), 65-67.

Labor is an important and crucial phase of pregnancy and hence, needs to be addressed scientifically. Basic neurological principles can be applied to the childbirth. The present study has used the principle of positive visualization along with the physical activity in the form of yoga to see the labor outcome. Ninety prim parous were selected with the method of randomization. They were matched of socio-economic status and health. The high-risk pregnancies were not included in the study. Ninety subjects were divided into three groups of thirty each. The three groups were Yoga Group, Yoga &Anupreksha Group, and Control Group. Yoga & Anupreksha Group was given contemplation for a normal delivery with short and easy labor. Yoga Group practiced only yoga and the Control Group was assigned thirty to forty-five minutes' walk. The results were very encouraging. The labor duration range dropped from 24 – 8 hours to 6 – 0.5 hours. The ratio of normal delivery went up drastically from 11 to 28.

10. **Authors**: Beddoe, A. E., Yang, C. P. P., Kennedy, H. P., Weiss, S. J., & Lee, K. A.

Title: The Effects of Mindfulness-Based Yoga During Pregnancy on Maternal Psychological and Physical Distress
Journal: *Journal of Obstetric, Gynecologic & Neonatal Nursing*, 2009, *38*(3), 310-319.
The feasibility and level of acceptability of a mindful yoga intervention provided during pregnancy and to gather preliminary data on the efficacy of the intervention in reducing distress. Baseline and post-treatment measures examined state and trait anxiety, perceived stress, pain, and morning salivary cortisol in a single treatment group. Post intervention data also included participant evaluation of the intervention. The 7 weeks mindfulness-based yoga group intervention combined elements of Iyengar yoga and mindfulness-based stress reduction. Sixteen healthy pregnant nulliparous women with singleton pregnancies between 12 and 32 weeks gestation at the time of enrollment. Outcomes were evaluated from pre- to postintervention and between second and third trimesters with repeated measures analysis of variance and post hoc nonparametric tests. Women practicing mindful yoga in their second trimester reported significant reductions in physical pain from baseline to postintervention compared with women in the third trimester whose pain increased. Women in their third trimester showed greater reductions

in perceived stress and trait anxiety. They concluded that preliminary evidence supports yoga's potential efficacy in these areas, particularly if started early in the pregnancy.

11. **Authors**: Chuntharapat, S., Petpichetchian, W., & Hatthakit, U.

Title: Yoga during pregnancy: Effects on maternal comfort, labor pain and birth outcomes

Journal: *Complementary therapies in clinical practice*, 2008, *14*(2), 105-115. This study examined the effects of a yoga program during pregnancy, on maternal comfort, labor pain, and birth outcomes. A randomized trial was conducted using 74-primigravid Thai women who were equally divided into two groups (experimental and control). The yoga program involved six, 1-h sessions at prescribed weeks of gestation. A variety of instruments were used to assess maternal comfort, labor pain and birth outcomes. The experimental group was found to have higher levels of maternal comfort during labor and 2 h post-labor, and experienced less subject evaluated labor pain than the control group. In each group, pain increased and maternal comfort decreased as labor progressed. No differences were found, between the groups, regarding pethidine usage, labor augmentation or newborn Apgar scores at 1 and 5 min. The experimental group was found to have a shorter duration of the first stage of labor, as well as the total time of labor.

12. **Authors**: Thakur, J.

Title: Yoga in pregnancy: a boon to motherhood

Journal: *Journal of Ayurveda and Holistic Medicine (JAHM)*, 2016, 3(6), 121-129.

Practicing yoga during pregnancy provides a great range of activity and benefits to unborn child and mother by numerous ways. Yoga soothes the mind, refocus the energy and prepare the woman physiologically and psychologically for labour. Different breathing techniques impart invaluable neuro-muscular control and helps in coordinated relaxation and contraction of uterus. Different type of asanas (postures),are described in Ayurveda and Yoga darshan texts which can be performed by a pregnant woman as they consume low energy and provide greater benefits. Published articles and different studies with references have been considered to support the effect of yoga in pregnancy. Yoga practicing includes physical postures and breathing techniques which minimizes the complication of pregnancy, like pregnancy induced hypertension, intrauterine growth retardation and pre-term delivery etc. Western exercises bring about what is known as phase contraction of muscles while yogic exercises create a static contraction which maintains a muscle under tension without causing repeated motions [1]. An approach to yoga in pregnancy can improve birth weight; decrease pre-term labour, decreased IUGR with least or no complications.

Exercise to Improve IQ

Exercise plays a major role in improving the IQ level of a fetus (Unborn baby in the womb). Low-impact exercises like walking and swimming improve the blood circulation and increased nutrient supply boosts the brain development. After five months of pregnancy, mother can rock gently and slowly in a rocking chair several times in a day. It is likely to enhance neuromotor development and coordination ability of the baby.

Reduce Stress:

The amount of stress the expecting mother may have during her pregnancy affects the development of the baby because chronic stress produces a hormone called cortisol which affects the baby. Some research indicates that high stress during pregnancy can result in lower intelligence quotient (IQ) scores, Pregnant women can try journal writing, taking plenty of naps, reading to the baby, soaking the feet for relaxation, meditation and yoga.

Stimulation

Babies have a biological need to learn. Any stimulation through his special senses of hearing, sight, taste, smell and touch provided during fetal life and preschool years have profound effect on the growth and maturation of brain. It has been shown that stimulation program can promote faster growth, improve coordination of muscular movements, increase span of concentration and raise the baby's IQ by as much as fifteen points. Hearing and touch are well developed for the baby in the womb.

Touch to boost up IQ

The miraculous power of touch for boosting IQ. Pregnant women can experience the movements of the baby from fifth month of pregnancy and by the seventh or eighth month the movements become very clear and the mother can feel the kick and jerks of the baby. If we keenly observe, we will notice certain parts of the baby such as feet, palm or head clearly over the abdomen. This is the best time we can connect with the baby in the womb as the baby can also feel the touch. This stimulates the baby's brain to search for more sensations and thus improves the sensory skills. Research also suggests that this type of stimulation is relaxing and reassuring for the baby. The baby will often respond to this stimulation by kicking or pushing back.

Nature Walk

Through the centuries, human beings have been drawn to nature to relax,

recuperate, and find temporary freedom from the stressors of everyday life. These ventures are based on the age-old belief in the salubrious effects of exposure to nature. Stress relief, escaping from civilization, clearing the head, reflecting on important life issues, experiencing beauty and connecting with nature are among the dominant self-reported motives. The single most important self-reported benefit of exposure to both nature-rich urban places and wilderness areas, however, is stress mitigation.

Restorative effects of nature exposure have been psychologically and physiologically accounted for in terms of "reduction in cognitive fatigue, decreased stress levels, increased focus, increased positive affect, decreased negative affect, and decreased sympathetic nervous system activity".

1. **Authors**: Olafsdottir, G., Cloke, P., Schulz, A., Van Dyck, Z., Eysteinsson, T., Thorleifsdottir, B., & Vögele, C.

Title: Health Benefits of Walking in Nature: A Randomized Controlled Study Under Conditions of Real-Life Stress

Journal: Environment and behaviour, 2020, 52(3), 248-274.

They investigated the effects of recreational exposure to the natural environment on mood and psychophysiological responses to stress. They hypothesized that walking in nature has restorative effects over and above the effects of exposure to nature scenes (viewing nature on TV) or physical exercise alone (walking on a treadmill in a gym) and that these effects are greater when participants were expected to be more stressed. Healthy university students ($N = 90$) were randomly allocated to one of three conditions and tested during an exam-free period and again during their exam time. Mood and psychophysiological responses were assessed before and after the interventions, and again after a laboratory stressor. All interventions had restorative effects on cortisol levels ($p < .001$), yet walking in nature resulted in lower cortisol levels than did nature viewing ($p < .05$) during the exam period. Walking in nature improved mood more than watching nature scenes ($p < .001$) or physical exercise alone ($p < .05$).

Religious beliefs

1. **Authors**: Aziato, L., Odai, P. N., & Omenyo, C. N.

    Title: Religious beliefs and practices in pregnancy and labour: an inductive qualitative study among post-partum women in Ghana

    Journal: *BMC pregnancy and childbirth*, 2016, *16*(1), 1-10.

    Religiosity in health care delivery has attracted some attention in contemporary literature. The religious beliefs and practices of patients play an important role in the recovery of the patient. Pregnant women and women in labour exhibit their faith and use religious artefacts. This phenomenon is poorly understood thus investigate the religious beliefs and practices of post-partum Ghanaian women. A descriptive phenomenological study was conducted inductively involving 13 women who were sampled purposively. Individual in-depth interviews were conducted in English, Ga, Twi and Ewe. The interviews were audio-taped and transcribed. Concurrent analysis was done employing the principles of content analysis. Ethical approval was obtained for the study and anonymity and confidentiality were ensured. Themes generated revealed religious beliefs and practices such as prayer, singing, thanksgiving at church, fellowship and emotional support. Pastors' spiritual interventions in pregnancy included prayer and revelations, reversing negative dreams, laying of hands and anointing women. Also, traditional beliefs and practices were food and water restrictions and tribal rituals. Religious artefacts used in pregnancy and labour were anointing oil, blessed water, sticker, blessed white handkerchief, blessed sand, Bible and Rosary. Family influence and secrecy were associated with the use of artefacts. They concluded that pregnant women and women in labour should be supported to exercise their religious beliefs and practices.

CHAPTER FOUR

DIET COUNSELLING AND PRENATAL EDUCATION

Pregnancy is a long period and includes many abnormal feelings and atypical taste developments also. But at the same time it is very important for the would-be mother to give the child developing in her womb a balanced diet on regular basis.

Pregnancy diet is a diet that is specially planned keeping in mind the well-being of the mother and the child. Everything has to be balanced and you also have to check out things at times. Food items that are rich in vitamins and minerals are essential for the pregnant woman. There is requirement of higher dose of certain vitamins and minerals. If this is not covered through pregnancy diet, they are prescribed dietary supplements. However, increase in servings of fruits and vegetables daily help pregnant women keep fit and it also protects the child from certain typical birth defects also.

Nutrition education and counselling (NEC) is a commonly applied strategy to improve maternal nutrition during pregnancy. However, with the exception special populations and specific diets, the effect of NEC on maternal, neonatal and child health outcomes has not been systematically reviewed.

1. **Authors**: Christian, P., Mullany, L. C., Hurley, K. M., Katz, J., & Black, R. E.

   Title: Nutrition and maternal, neonatal, and child health
   Journal: Seminars in perinatology, 2015, (Vol. 39, No. 5, pp. 361-372). WB Saunders.

   The central role of nutrition in advancing the maternal, newborn, and child health agenda with a focus on evidence for effective interventions generated using randomized controlled trials in low-and middle-income countries (LMIC). The 1000 days spanning from conception to 2 years of life area critical period of time when nutritional needs must be ensured can lead to adverse impacts on short-term survival as well as long- term health and development. The burden of maternal mortality continues to be high in many under-resourced settings; prenatal calcium supplementation in populations with low intakes can reduce the risk of pre-eclampsia and eclampsia morbidity and mortality and is recommended, and antenatal iron folic acid use in many countries may reduce anemia, a condition that may be an underlying factor in postpartum hemorrhage. Sufficient evidence exists to promote multiple micronutrient supplementations during pregnancy to reduce fetal growth restriction and low birth weight.

1. **Authors**: Pooja, B., Pradeep, K., Niraj, S., & Varsha, S.

Title: Effect of Garbhini Ahara-Vihara (Diet & Lifestyle in Pregnancy) On Garbhastha Sishu (Fetus) and Offspring.

Journal: *Indian Journal of Public Health Research & Development*, 2020, *11*(6), 152-156.

Fetal growth is dependent on appropriate diet and life style of pregnant mother. Organogenesis is that period when important organ of fetus are developing. It is 6-10 wks of intrauterine life. During this period fetus is most at risk from birth defects caused by external factors. Many diseases and fetal development disorders are consider as being related to prenatal exposure to endocrine disrupting chemicals (EDC). The physical, mental, social, and spiritual well-being during pregnancy and practice of a wholesome regimen, play a prime role in achieving a healthy progeny.

3. **Authors**: Chen, X., Zhao, D., Mao, X., Xia, Y., Baker, P. N., & Zhang, H. **Title**: Maternal Dietary Patterns and Pregnancy Outcome

Journal: Nutrients 2016, 8, 351;

The studies detailed above highlight the importance of emphasising healthy dietary choices in preconception counseling to optimise not only reproductive outcomes but also general maternal health. Current guidelines of preconception care emphasise that nutrition and certain lifestyle factors play an important role in pregnancy. This review finds evidence that, for European countries, the Mediterranean diet is a relatively healthy diet. Importantly, the diets with higher intake of fruits, vegetables, legumes and fish have positive pregnancy outcomes in general and this conclusive evidence should be communicated to women specifically. As a modifiable factor, diet is a key area for intervention in pregnant women, but the precise content of the intervention is yet to be elucidated.

4. **Authors**: Girard, A. W., & Olude, O.

Title: Nutrition Education and Counselling Provided during Pregnancy: Effects on Maternal, Neonatal and Child Health Outcomes

Journal: *Paediatric and perinatal epidemiology*, 2012, 26, 191-204.

Nutrition education and counselling (NEC) is a commonly applied strategy to improve maternal nutrition during pregnancy. However, with the exception special populations and specific diets, the effect of NEC on maternal, neonatal and child health outcomes has not been systematically reviewed. They conducted meta-analyses for the effect of NEC on maternal, neonatal and infant health outcomes including gestational weight gain, maternal anaemia, birthweight, low birthweight and preterm delivery. NEC significantly improved gestational weight gain by 0.45 kg, reduced the risk of anaemia in late pregnancy by 30%, increased birth weight by 105 g and lowered the risk of preterm delivery by 19%. The effect of NEC on risk of low birth weight was not significant. The effect of NEC was greater when provided with nutrition support, for example, food or micronutrient supplements or nutrition safety nets. The overall quality of the body of evidence was deemed low for all outcomes due to high heterogeneity, poor study designs and other biases. Additional well designed research that is grounded in appropriate theories of behaviour change is needed to improve confidence in the effect of NEC.

5. **Authors**: Garg, A., & Kashyap, S.

Title: Effect of counseling on nutritional status during pregnancy

Journal: *The Indian Journal of Pediatrics*, 2006, 73(8), 687-692.

Hundred pregnant women belonging to low socio-economic status were interviewed. Based on lacune, nutrition education (NE) was given in the form of simple messages to 50 subjects (NE-group) over 10–16 weeks period, while the remaining 50 formed the comparison group (Non-NE group). Tools used were individual counselling, weekly home visits and group meetings. Anthropometric measurements taken were height and weight. Dietary data was collected using 24-hour recall and food frequency questionnaire. Haemoglobin estimation was done. Effect of intervention was assessed by monitoring changes in dietary practices, weight gain, and nutritional status of the subjects. They found low mean maternal body weight (51.05±7.26 kg), 96.3% anemia prevalence and severely suboptimal dietary intakes. Post-NE results revealed a significant increase in quality and quantity of the diets consumed. Mean hemoglobin levels significantly increased (Post-NE*vs* Non-NE=9.65±0.97*vs* 7.85±1.58, p<0.001) and anemia prevalence reduced (Post-NE*vs* Non-NE=78.7%*vs* 96%) in post-NE group. They concluded that individual counselling with weekly reinforcement can bring about improvement in nutritional status during pregnancy.

6. **Authors**: Lindsay, K. L., Buss, C., Wadhwa, P. D., & Entringer, S.

Title: The Interplay between Maternal Nutrition and Stress during Pregnancy:
Issues and Considerations
Journal: *Annals of Nutrition and Metabolism*, 2017, *70*(3), 191-200.

During pregnancy, maternal psychosocial stress, dietary behavior, and nutritional state likely regulate and counter-regulate one another. Emerging evidence suggests that omega-3 fatty acids may attenuate maternal psychosocial stress, and that high maternal pre-pregnancy body mass index exacerbates unhealthy dietary behaviors under high-stress conditions. Longitudinal studies are warranted in order to understand the interplay between prenatal psychosocial stress, diet, and stress- and nutrition-related biomarkers to obtain further insight and inform the development and design of future, more effective intervention trials for improved maternal and child health outcomes.

7. **Authors**: Ramakrishnan, U., Grant, F., Goldenberg, T., Zongrone, A., & Martorell, R.

Title: Effect of Women's Nutrition before and during Early Pregnancy on Maternal and Infant Outcomes: A Systematic Review
Journal: *Paediatric and perinatal epidemiology*, 2012, *26*, 285-301.

Intervention trials and observational studies show that periconceptional (<12 weeks gestation) folic acid supplementation significantly reduced the risk of neural tube defects. Observational studies suggest that preconceptional and periconceptional intake of vitamin and mineral supplements is associated with a reduced risk of delivering offspring who are low birth weight and/or small-for gestational age (SGA) and preterm deliveries (PTD). Some studies report that indicators of maternal prepregnancy size, low stature, underweight and overweight are associated with increased risks of PTD and SGA. The available data indicate the importance of women's nutrition prior to and during the first trimester of pregnancy, but there is a need for well-designed prospective studies and controlled trials in developing country settings that examine relationships with low birthweight, SGA, PTD, stillbirth and maternal and neonatal mortality. The knowledge gaps that need to be addressed include the evaluation of periconceptional interventions such as food supplements, multivitamin-mineral supplements and/or specific micronutrients (iron, zinc, iodine, vitamin B-6 and B-12) as well as the relationship between measures of prepregnancy body size and composition and maternal, neonatal and child health outcomes.

8. **Authors**: Yang, Z., & Huffman, S. L.

Title: Nutrition in pregnancy and early childhood and associations with obesity in developing countries
Journal: *Maternal & child nutrition*, 2013, 9, 105-119.
Obesity is an increasing problem in developing countries, and finding means to reduce it is essential. Improving maternal, infant and young child nutrition is an approach that will have multiple health benefits in addition to reducing obesity in adulthood. Adequate and balanced

protein, energy and micronutrient intakes during pregnancy might be a protective factor for adult obesity. Improving women's nutritional status prior to and during pregnancy can substantially reduce the risk of low birthweight. Low birthweight appeared to have less lean body mass, lower BMI and greater fat mass in adults.

9. **Authors**: Bahrami, N., Simbar, M., & Bahrami, S.

Title: The Effect of Prenatal Education on Mother's Quality of Life during First Year Postpartum among Iranian Women: A Randomized Controlled Trial

Journal: *International journal of fertility & sterility*, 2013, 7(3), 169.

Antenatal educations provide information regarding pregnancy, birth, infant care and early parenthood. The purpose of this study was to determine effect of prenatal education on mother's quality of life during first year after childbirth among Iranian women. This single-blind randomized control trial study was performed on 160 first-time pregnant women; with a singleton fetus; aged 18 to 35; without history of medical, psychological, and infertility diseases; as well as with at least eight prenatal visits during pregnancy. Participants were invited into two groups of intervention (n=80) and control (n=80). The antenatal education classes were consisted of eight sessions, and then, mother's quality of life was evaluated during first year after childbirth. Data was analyzed using t test, chi-square, and Mann-Withney. The interventional group demonstrated higher scores of quality of life domains than the control group (p<0.05). The interventional group (at one year postpartum) demonstrated significantly higher scores for quality of life in the physical health, psychological health, and environmental health domains compared to the control group. In addition, the interventional group showed a significant increase in the mean scores for the domains of physical, psychological, and environmental health from 6-8 weeks to 1 year postpartum. The study showed that women receiving prenatal education had higher level of happiness and satisfaction in their overall quality of life and health, respectively.

10. **Authors:** Rahimi, F., Islami, F., & Kahangi, M. M.

Title: Effects of Prenatal Education on Maternal and Neonatal Outcomes in High Risk Pregnant Women

Journal: *Pajouhan Scientific Journal*, 2018, 16(3), 48-57.

Lack of awareness and the fear of women is one of the reasons for cesarean delivery and the occurrence of complications in maternal and neonatal period in our country. This study was conducted to investigate the effect of prenatal education on maternal and neonatal outcomes in high risk pregnant women. The study was done as a randomized clinical trial on 150 high risk pregnant women was referred to Amiralmomenin Hospital in Shahreza, Iran in 2014. Samples were randomly assigned to control and intervention groups. The control group only received routine pregnancy care and case group received routine pregnancy care and prenatal education. After delivery, Maternal and neonatal outcomes including type of delivery, Apgar index, weight and height, head circumference, and jaundice were assessed by using Chi-square and independent t-test. Intervention and control groups did not significant in terms of demographic and obstetric variables (P>0/05). The results showed that a significant difference between two groups in type of delivery, height, weight and head circumference (P<0/001). However there was no significant difference between the two groups in Apgar scores and in jaundice (P>0.05). They concluded that raising awareness and education of pregnant women during pregnancy promote and improve the health of the baby and be a natural delivery. Therefore, it is suggested that prenatal education more widely used.

11. **Authors**: Yikar, S. K., & Nazik, E.

Title: Effects of prenatal education on complaints during pregnancy and on quality of life.

Journal: *Patient education and counseling, 102*(1), 119-125.

This study is a quasi-experimental research with a control group. Personal Information Form and Scale of Complaints during Pregnancy and their Effects on Quality of Life (SCPEQL) were used to collect the data. Thirty participants were included in both the control and the intervention groups ($N = 60$). They found that the mean scores of SCPEQL of the intervention group was 46.2 ± 21.1 and the mean scores of SCPEQL of the control group was 99.8 ± 21.6 in 2nd trimester. In the 3rd trimester, the mean score of SCPEQL of the intervention group was 43.5 ± 16.4, and the mean score of SCPEQL of the control group was 108.0 ± 16.8. The difference between the groups was statistically significant in 2nd and 3rd trimesters ($p < 0.05$). Findings of the study suggest that providing prenatal education reduces complaints and increases quality of life of pregnant women.

12. **Authors**: Agbeno, E. K., Gbagbo, F. Y., Morhe, E. S. K., Maltima, S. I., & Sarbeng, K.

Title: Pregnancy options counselling in Ghana: a case study of women with unintended pregnancies in Kumasi metropolis, Ghana

Journal: *BMC pregnancy and childbirth*, 2019, *19*(1), 1-9.

Analytical cross-sectional study design was done in selected specialised public and NGO health facilities within Kumasi Metropolis of Ghana, using self-administered structured questionnaires for data collection from 1st January to 30th April, 2014. Participants were 442 women with unintended pregnancies seeking abortion services. Data was analysed using Epi-Info (7.1.1.14) and STATA 12 to generate descriptive statistics, Pearson chi-square and multivariable logistic regressions. They found that respondents had divergent reproductive and socio-demographic profiles. Majority (about 58%) of them had been pregnant more than twice, but about 53% of this population had no biological children. (Although about 90% of respondents held perceptions that the index and previous pregnancies were mistimed/unintended, the majority (72%) had no induced abortion history. Induced abortion (208,49%) and parenting (216,51%) were mentioned as the only available options to unintended pregnancy in hospitals. Exposure to options counselling was observed to be significantly associated with parity (P=< 0.001), gestational age (P=< 0.001), previous induced abortions (P=< 0.001), perception of pregnancy at conception (P=<0.001) and level of education (P=0.002). The logistic regression analysis also shows that higher education has statistically significant effect on being exposed to options counselling (P=< 0.001). Majority of respondents (95%) were not aware that giving a child up for adoption is an option to abortion in Ghana. They concluded that pregnancy options counselling remains a major challenge in comprehensive abortion care in Ghana. Although higher educational attainments significantly expose women to options counselling for informed decisions, the less educated are disadvantaged in this regard. Further research on type and depth of counselling services provided to pregnant women in health facilities is required to inform health policy and program decisions.

13. **Authors**: Elsinga, J., de Jong-Potjer, L. C., van der Pal-de, K. M., le Cessie, S., Assendelft, W. J., & Buitendijk, S. E.

Title: The Effect Of Preconception Counselling On Lifestyle And Other Behaviour Before And During Pregnancy

Journal: *Women's Health Issues*, 2008, *18*(6), S117-S125.

They conducted a randomized controlled trial, "Parents to Be." with this study, they sought to assess the extent to which women who have participated in preconception counselling (PCC) increase their knowledge on pregnancy-related risk factors and preventive measures and change their behaviour before and during pregnancy and to provide an overview of adverse pregnancy outcomes among such women. Knowledge: Women aged 18–40 who attended PCC and women who received standard care were matched on previous pregnancy, time since last pregnancy, age, country of birth and educational achievement. They were sent a questionnaire on knowledge about pregnancy related risk factors and preventive measures. Behaviour: Data on pregnancies and outcomes were collected. Two months after pregnancy, a questionnaire was sent regarding behaviour before and during pregnancy. They found knowledge of women who received PCC (81.5%; n 211) exceeded that of women who did not (76.9%; n 422). Levels of knowledge in women who were not yet pregnant after PCC were comparable to those in women who became pregnant after PCC, indicating that, even before pregnancy, PCC increased knowledge in women contemplating pregnancy. After PCC, significantly more women started using folic acid before pregnancy and reduced alcohol use during the first 3 months of pregnancy). Among the group receiving standard care, about 20% of all pregnancies ended in an adverse outcome; in the group with PCC this was 16%. They concluded after PCC, women have more knowledge about essential items. Importantly, they gained this greater knowledge before pregnancy and more women changed their behaviour to reduce adverse pregnancy outcomes.

<u>Story time with baby</u>

Reading stories aloud to the baby during pregnancy has advantages, it is a useful bonding experience. It also encourages the cognitive development of the baby. Pregnant women need to choose a relaxing and quiet place and suitable time and make it a daily routine. They can select stories from scriptures, verses, autobiographies of great people, moral stories which they can tell again as bed time stories when the baby grows up. Choosing books that utilize repetition, rhyming, and rhythm can help to stimulate cognitive development, pattern recognition, and language skills in the children.

CHAPTER FIVE

ART BASED ACTIVITY

The transition to motherhood is a dynamic experience. Antenatal care and education are designed to support women during pregnancy; however childbearing women often report a further need for emotional and social support beyond preparation for birth. Broadening routine antenatal care to included art-based interventions may offer women an opportunity to explore important aspects of the transition to motherhood.

The concept of creativity and its application through various artistic and spiritual activities has been identified as a powerful catalyst for personal growth and emotional and spiritual adjustment in a range of life domains. Premised on the act of making, creativity underpins the conception of meaningful products and ideas through the convergence of cognitive and emotional processes, which in its optimal state, strengthens the human spirit and facilitates the natural healing process in the human psyche.

1. **Authors**: Crane, T., Buultjens, M., & Fenner, P.

Title: Art-based interventions during pregnancy to support women's wellbeing: An integrative review

Journal: *Women and Birth*, 2020.

Art-based engagements supported women to express complex emotion, fostered a sense of connection and strengthened personal resourcefulness. Creative expression provided an opportunity to explore important aspects of the motherhood experience including, complex emotion, identity and bonding with the unborn child. Being in a group enhanced the health effects of art-making and the social connection felt supportive when role and identity was evolving. They concluded whilst research on the current topic is emergent, preliminary results suggest that facilitated art-based programs are valuable for pregnant women. Art-based experiences offer women a unique opportunity to explore the full dimensionality of the transition to motherhood which can contribute to improved health and wellbeing. These findings suggest that art-based programs may serve to complement existing antenatal care models.

Art-based programs can offer pregnant women an important opportunity to explore broader dimensions of the transition to motherhood, which enhances health and improves wellbeing. Given the substantial and enduring impact of maternal distress on women and their families, the pressing need to continuously strive to improve the way in which women are supported in the transition to motherhood remains. The potential health enhancing and supportive role that art-based expression can play in a woman's life as she becomes a mother may go some way in providing women with an opportunity to express dimensions of the maternal experience that are outside the scope of verbal exchange and current antenatal care services. Exploring the possibility of complementing antenatal care for women who become mothers with creative, art-based groups is warranted.

CHAPTER SIX

BIBLIOGRAPHY

1. Agbeno, E. K., Gbagbo, F. Y., Morhe, E. S. K., Maltima, S. I., & Sarbeng, K. (2019). Pregnancy options counselling in Ghana: a case study of women with unintended pregnancies in Kumasi metropolis, Ghana. *BMC pregnancy and childbirth*, *19*(1), 1-9.

2. Agrawal, T., & Gupta, P. K. (2018). Garbhasanskar–A boon to get supraja. *The Pharma Innovation Journal*, *7*(6), 454-456.

3. Akmeşe, Z. B., & Oran, N. T. (2014). Effects of progressive muscle relaxation exercises accompanied by music on low back pain and quality of life during pregnancy. *Journal of midwifery & women's health*, *59*(5), 503-509.

4. Arya, R., Chansoria, M., Konanki, R., & Tiwari, D. K. (2012). Maternal music exposure during pregnancy influences neonatal behaviour: An open-label randomized controlled trial. *International journal of pediatrics*, *2012*.

5. Aziato, L., Odai, P. N., & Omenyo, C. N. (2016). Religious beliefs and practices in pregnancy and labour:

an inductive qualitative study among post-partum women in Ghana. *BMC pregnancy and childbirth, 16*(1), 1-10.

6. Bahrami, N., Simbar, M., & Bahrami, S. (2013). The effect of prenatal education on mother's quality of life during first year postpartum among iranian women: a randomized controlled trial. *International journal of fertility & sterility, 7*(3), 169.

7. Beddoe, A. E., Yang, C. P. P., Kennedy, H. P., Weiss, S. J., & Lee, K. A. (2009). The effects of mindfulness-based yoga during pregnancy on maternal psychological and physical distress. *Journal of Obstetric, Gynecologic & Neonatal Nursing, 38*(3), 310-319.

8. Beddoe, A. E., Yang, C. P. P., Kennedy, H. P., Weiss, S. J., & Lee, K. A. (2009). The effects of mindfulness-based yoga during pregnancy on maternal psychological and physical distress. *Journal of Obstetric, Gynecologic & Neonatal Nursing, 38*(3), 310-319.

9. Chang, H. C., Yu, C. H., Chen, S. Y., & Chen, C. H. (2015). The effects of music listening on psychosocial stress and maternal–fetal attachment during pregnancy. *Complementary therapies in medicine, 23*(4), 509-515.

10. Chang, M. Y., Chen, C. H., & Huang, K. F. (2008). Effects of music therapy on psychological health of women during pregnancy. *Journal of clinical nursing, 17*(19), 2580-2587.

11. Chaudhary, I., & Joshi, B. Efficacy of Blessings Meditation as a Behavioral Medicine in Enhancing Pregnancy Happiness. *Age (years), 20*(25), 18.

12. Chen, X., Zhao, D., Mao, X., Xia, Y., Baker, P. N., & Zhang, H. (2016). Maternal dietary patterns and pregnancy outcome. *Nutrients, 8*(6), 351.

13. Christian, P., Mullany, L. C., Hurley, K. M., Katz, J., & Black, R. E. (2015, August). Nutrition and maternal, neonatal, and child health. In *Seminars in perinatology* (Vol. 39, No. 5, pp. 361-372). WB Saunders.

14. Chuntharapat, S., Petpichetchian, W., & Hatthakit, U. (2008). Yoga during pregnancy: effects on maternal comfort, labor pain and birth outcomes. *Complementary therapies in clinical practice, 14*(2), 105-115.

15. Chuntharapat, S., Petpichetchian, W., & Hatthakit, U. (2008). Yoga during pregnancy: effects on maternal comfort, labor pain and birth outcomes. *Complementary therapies in clinical practice, 14*(2), 105-115.

16. Crane, T., Buultjens, M., & Fenner, P. (2020). Art-based interventions during pregnancy to support women's wellbeing: An integrative review. *Women and Birth.*

17. Dhapola, M. S., & Prasad, M. R. K. (2018). Role of different asanas during prenatal and postnatal pregnancy. *International Journal of Physical Education and Sports, 3*(12), 9-16.

18. Elsinga, J., de Jong-Potjer, L. C., van der Pal-de, K. M., le Cessie, S., Assendelft, W. J., & Buitendijk, S. E. (2008). The effect of preconception counselling on lifestyle and other behaviour before and during pregnancy. *Women's Health Issues, 18*(6), S117-S125.

19. Fritz, T. H., Ciupek, M., Kirkland, A., Ihme, K., Guha, A., Hoyer, J., & Villringer, A. (2014). Enhanced response to music in pregnancy. *Psychophysiology, 51*(9), 905-911.

20. García González, J., Ventura Miranda, M. I., Requena Mullor, M., Parron Carreño, T., & Alarcón Rodriguez, R. (2018). Effects of prenatal music stimulation on state/ trait anxiety in full-term pregnancy and its influence on childbirth: a randomized controlled trial. *The journal of maternal-fetal & neonatal medicine, 31*(8), 1058-1065.

21. Garg, A., & Kashyap, S. (2006). Effect of counseling on nutritional status during pregnancy. *The Indian Journal of Pediatrics, 73*(8), 687-692.

22. Girard, A. W., & Olude, O. (2012). Nutrition education and counselling provided during pregnancy: effects on maternal, neonatal and child health outcomes. *Paediatric and perinatal epidemiology, 26*, 191-204.

23. Gupta, A., Janu, N., & Punia, R. (2018). Efficacy of Yoga & Anupreksha in Natural Birthing and Reducing Labor Duration. Journal Of Humanities And Social Science (IOSR-JHSS), 23(4), 65-67.

24. Lindsay, K. L., Buss, C., Wadhwa, P. D., & Entringer, S. (2017). The interplay between maternal nutrition and stress during pregnancy: Issues and considerations. *Annals of Nutrition and Metabolism, 70*(3), 191-200.

25. Narendran, S., Nagarathna, R., Narendran, V., Gunasheela, S., & Nagendra, H. R. R. (2005). Efficacy of yoga on pregnancy outcome. *Journal of Alternative & Complementary Medicine, 11*(2), 237-244.

26. Nwebube, C., Glover, V., & Stewart, L. (2017). Prenatal listening to songs composed for pregnancy and symptoms of anxiety and depression: a pilot study. *BMC complementary and alternative medicine, 17*(1), 1-5.

27. Olafsdottir, G., Cloke, P., Schulz, A., Van Dyck, Z., Eysteinsson, T., Thorleifsdottir, B., & Vögele, C. (2020). Health benefits of walking in nature: A randomized controlled study under conditions of real-life stress. *Environment and Behavior, 52*(3), 248-274.

28. Pithadiya, A. C., Makwana, D., & Tomar, S. (2016). Garbhasanskar-A Technique Of Educating Foetus. *Pharma Science Monitor, 7*(1), 50-56

29. Pithadiya, A. C., Makwana, D., & Tomar, S. (2016). Garbhasanskar-A Technique Of Educating Foetus.

Pharma Science Monitor, 7(1), 50-56

30. Pithadiya, A. C., Makwana, D., & Tomar, S. (2016). Garbhasanskar-A Technique Of Educating Foetus. *Pharma Science Monitor, 7*(1), 50-56

31. Pooja, B., Pradeep, K., Niraj, S., & Varsha, S. (2020). Effect of Garbhini Ahara-Vihara (Diet & Lifestyle in Pregnancy) On Garbhastha Sishu (Fetus) and Offspring. *Indian Journal of Public Health Research & Development, 11*(6), 152-156.

32. Rahimi, F., Islami, F., & Kahangi, M. M. (2018). Effects of prenatal education on maternal and neonatal outcomes in high risk pregnant women. *Pajouhan Scientific Journal, 16*(3), 48-57.

33. Ramakrishnan, U., Grant, F., Goldenberg, T., Zongrone, A., & Martorell, R. (2012). Effect of women's nutrition before and during early pregnancy on maternal and infant outcomes: a systematic review. *Paediatric and perinatal epidemiology, 26*, 285-301.

34. Surucu, S. G., Ozturk, M., Vurgec, B. A., Alan, S., & Akbas, M. (2018). The effect of music on pain and anxiety of women during labour on first time pregnancy: A study from Turkey. *Complementary therapies in clinical practice, 30*, 96-102.

35. Tejwani, N., Roy, P. K., & Mishra, R. (2013). Role Of Yoga For Better Outcome Of Pregnancy. *National Journal of Integrated Research in Medicine, 4*(4).

36. Thakur, J. (2016). Yoga in pregnancy: A boon to motherhood. *Journal of Ayurveda and Holistic Medicine (JAHM), 3*(6), 121-129.

37. Wulff, V., Hepp, P., Wolf, O. T., Balan, P., Hagenbeck, C., Fehm, T., & Schaal, N. K. (2021). The effects of a music and singing intervention during pregnancy on maternal well-being and mother–infant bonding: a randomised,

controlled study. *Archives of gynecology and obstetrics, 303*(1), 69-83.

38. Yang, Z., & Huffman, S. L. (2013). Nutrition in pregnancy and early childhood and associations with obesity in developing countries. *Maternal & child nutrition, 9,* 105-119.

Yikar, S. K., & Nazik, E. (2019). Effects of prenatal education on complaints during pregnancy and on quality of life. *Patient education and counseling, 102*(1), 119-125.